HEALING FIBROIDS

A Self-Care Handbook for Uterine Wellness and Balance

ACHIENG ORETA

Copyright © 2024

Disclaimer

Healing Fibroids: A Self-Care Handbook for Uterine Wellness and Balance is an offering to support you with self-care practices that can work alongside medical treatment. This book shares ideas and information from public sources and isn't a replacement for medical advice. Be sure to talk with your healthcare provider for guidance that's right for you. Wishing your health, balance, and peace on your journey to wellness.

TABLE OF CONTENT

Introduction………………………………………….............5

Chapter 1 The Sacred Nature of The Uterus………….....6

Chapter 2 Understanding Fiibroids……………………...9

Chapter 3 Nourishing Your Womb Through Food... 13

Chapter 4 The Importance of Vitamin D …………….....17

Chapter 5 Stress and Fibroids ……………….………....22

Chapter 6 Physical Movement and Womb Health…..... 27

Chapter 7 Rest and Recovery for Womb Health……....30

Chapter 8 The Benefits of Herbal Teas………..……….34

Chapter 9 Cleaning Living……………………………....40

Chapter 10 Emotional Healing………………………….50

Chapter 11 Evocation………………………………....54

References……………………………………………59

INTRODUTION

Living with fibroids had been a deeply challenging and stressful experience. My desire to heal drove me to seek support across continents. From consulting doctors in the United States to finding care in Kisumu, Kenya, I remained open to exploring any path that could bring relief. Along the way, I discovered that simple healthy habits, like eating organic foods and spending time in the sun, became essential for my overall well-being, especially for the health of my uterus. The tips and information in this book are drawn from my own experiences and publicly available resources I've gathered along the way. While there is so much more out there, I'm sharing this as an act of gratitude for my own wellness journey, with the hope that it might support you too. Some of these self-care practices may resonate with you, while others may not—and that's perfectly okay. I encourage you to take what feels right for you and, most importantly, to discuss any new practices with your healthcare provider. Remember to do your own research to find the best approach for your unique body and health journey. My hope is that this book becomes a source of inspiration and support as you move toward greater wellness. Happy Healing!

CHAPTER 1

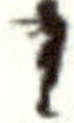

THE SACRED NATURE OF THE UTERUS

Have you ever considered that your uterus, or womb space, is more than just an organ designed for childbirth and monthly periods? Beyond its biological functions, the womb is a powerful energetic center, capable of creating not only physical life but also manifesting your dreams, desires, and intentions. Across many ancient cultures, the womb has been revered as the seat of feminine power—a portal of transformation on physical, spiritual, and energetic levels

In the spirituality of Ancient Kemet, the goddess Hathor symbolized fertility and the divine feminine, honoring the womb as a portal for physical and spiritual transformation. Today, many holistic practices support this ancient wisdom. In *Sacred Woman,* Queen Afua explores the womb as a sacred space that connects women to their spiritual power and life purpose. She views it as a gateway for healing and transformation. (Afua, 2001). Similarly, Tami Lynn Kent, in *The Wild Feminine*, emphasizes the womb as an energetic center for creativity and healing, encouraging women to reconnect with this vital source of feminine power. (Kent, 2011).

The womb's magnetism works by drawing in energies that resonate with your truest desires. Physically, it nurtures sperm to create life, mirroring its energetic ability to attract and hold intentions. However, just as it can nurture life, the womb may also absorb unresolved emotions, unmet needs, and deeply rooted beliefs. These unresolved patterns can sometimes manifest as physical conditions, such as fibroids. This notion is supported by some holistic health practitioners, such as Dr. Christiane Northrup, who suggests that fibroids are thought to symbolize unresolved emotional patterns or imbalances that call for healing (Northrup, 2010

To align the womb's magnetism with your highest good, it's essential to cultivate a strong, loving connection with it. Think of your womb as a home—keeping it clean, both physically and energetically, helps maintain balance. When the womb is overwhelmed, imbalance may arise, manifesting as physical issues like heavy blood flow, which can lead to energy drains, missed opportunities, and blocked abundance in other areas of life, such as relationships or work.

Caring for your womb can also deepen your intuition and bring your dreams to life. For instance, if you're aiming to land a new job or attract clients to your business, you can connect with your womb as a source of creative energy. As Tami Lynn Kent explains, the womb is not just a physical organ; it is a wellspring of creativity and intuition. Intentional self-care creates inner balance, which helps you trust yourself and take purposeful steps forward.

If you're wondering how to use your womb as a center for manifesting your desires, start with a simple practice. Place your hands over your lower abdomen, take a few deep breaths, and set an intention. Hold this intention and say an affirmation, either aloud or in your mind. For example: "I am open to womb healing. My womb is a space of health, harmony, and balance." or "My heart and womb invite and support relationships that are loving and true." As you do this, picture light radiating from your womb, carrying your intention out into the universe. When you're ready, close the practice with gratitude.

Incorporating supportive rituals like womb steaming, belly massages, or drinking herbal teas such as mugwort, known for its clarity-enhancing properties, can deepen this connection. Consistency is key. The more you nurture your connection with your womb, the more you'll unlock its powerful energy. Explore practices that feel right for you and honor your unique journey.

CHAPTER 2

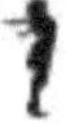

UNDERSTANDING FIBROIDS?

Fibroids, also known as uterine fibroids or leiomyomas, are non-cancerous growths that develop in or around the uterus. Composed of muscle and connective tissue, these growths often appear during a woman's reproductive years. While fibroids are benign, they can sometimes cause symptoms like heavy menstrual bleeding, pelvic pain, and fertility challenges. In certain cases, they can grow large enough to cause significant discomfort (U.S. Department of Health and Human Services, 2024).

Different Types of Fibroids.

Fibroids grow in different areas of the uterus, and their location determines their type:

Intramural Fibroids: These grow within the muscular wall of the uterus and are the most common type.

Subserosal Fibroids: Found on the outer wall of the uterus, they can press on nearby organs, causing discomfort.

Submucosal Fibroids: Located just under the uterine lining, these can lead to heavy bleeding and may affect fertility.

Pedunculated Fibroids: These grow on a stalk, either inside or outside the uterus (U.S. Department of Health and Human Services, 2024).

Symptoms of Fibroids

Fibroid symptoms vary depending on their size, number, and location. Some women may have no symptoms, while others experience significant discomfort. Common symptoms include:

Heavy or Prolonged Menstrual Bleeding: Often associated with submucosal fibroids, this can increase the risk of anemia (Parker, 2007).

Pelvic Pain and Pressure: Larger fibroids can create feelings of fullness, bloating, or abdominal discomfort (Stewart, 2015).

Frequent Urination: Fibroids pressing on the bladder can lead to frequent urination or difficulty fully emptying the bladder (Parker, 2007).

Lower Back Pain: Fibroids located toward the back of the uterus may cause back pain (Vollenhoven, 1998).

Pain During Intercourse: Fibroids near the cervix or within the uterus can result in discomfort during sex (Stewart, 2015).

Constipation: Larger fibroids pressing on the rectum can make bowel movements difficult (Parker, 2007).

Enlarged Abdomen: In some cases, fibroids grow large

enough to cause abdominal enlargement, resembling pregnancy (Stewart, 2015).

Fertility Issues: Submucosal fibroids growing within the uterine cavity may interfere with conception or increase the risk of miscarriage (Vollenhoven, 1998).

Factors Influencing Fibroid Development

Fibroid growth is influenced by genetics, hormones, environmental factors, and lifestyle choices.

Genetic Factors: The Role of the MED12 Gene

Research suggests that genetic mutations, particularly in the MED12 gene, significantly contribute to fibroid development. This gene regulates cell growth in the uterus's smooth muscle. When mutated, it can lead to abnormal cell division and fibroid formation. These mutations are commonly found in intramural and subserosal fibroids, which may explain why women with a family history are more prone to developing fibroids (Taylor & Parrott, 2023).).

Hormonal Influences

Hormonal imbalances, especially elevated levels of estrogen and progesterone, are strongly linked to fibroid growth. These hormones promote the growth of uterine cells, increasing the likelihood of fibroids in women with high hormone levels.

Environmental Factors

Environmental factors also play a role. Endocrine-disrupting chemicals (EDCs), such as phthalates, BPA, and parabens, found in plastics, personal care products, and other items, mimic estrogen and disrupt hormonal balance. These chemicals may contribute to fibroid growth in genetically predisposed women, amplifying hormonal imbalances (Baird & Patisaul, 2021).

Self-Care Tips If You Suspect Fibroids

Get a Medical Checkup: If you experience abnormal bleeding or any fibroid-related symptoms mentioned above, consult a healthcare provider.

Educate Yourself: Learn about fibroids, their causes, and treatment options. Open conversations with your doctor can help you better understand your condition.

Understand Your Hormones: Familiarize yourself with the role of estrogen and progesterone in fibroid growth. Consider hormone-balancing practices such as maintaining a healthy diet and reducing stress. Consult your doctor about supplements that may help.

Reduce Chemicals Exposure: Choose beauty and personal care products free of endocrine-disrupting chemicals, such as parabens and phthalates, to minimize their impact on hormonal balance (Baird & Patisaul, 2021).

CHAPTER 3

HOW DIET AFFECTS YOUR WOMB

As mentioned in Chapter 1, your womb is a sacred center of creative energy and a vessel for manifestation. The foods you eat can either amplify this creative force and enhance its magnetic power or stifle its flow. Your diet is an opportunity to align with the energies of healing, balance, and abundance. Eating whole, organic, and nutrient-rich foods supports the vitality of your womb. Because whole foods are naturally abundant, the energy of abundance flows effortlessly through your body. A healthy diet benefits not only your physical health but also your energetic vibration.

Eat organic: When I focused on improving my womb health, I discovered the transformative power of food. One of the first changes I made was committing fully to an organic diet. Although I occasionally chose organic foods before, I sometimes switched back to conventional options. But when I went fully organic, I noticed less bloating, less discomfort, and an energizing shift in how I felt overall. Eating organic felt like welcoming the Earth's pure energy into my body. Research shows that organic foods reduce exposure to pesticides and chemicals, which can support hormonal balance and reproductive health (*Smith-Spangler et al., 2012*).

True organic foods are grown without synthetic pesticides, herbicides, or genetically modified organisms. These practices support soil health and biodiversity. To ensure you're choosing genuine organic produce, look for the USDA Organic label or a five-digit PLU code starting with "9" (U.S. Department of Agriculture, 2023). Shopping at farmers' markets and local co-ops is another great way to find fresh, authentically organic foods. For more in-depth guidance, *Eating on the Wild Side* by Jo Robinson offers valuable insights on choosing between organic and conventional options.

Reducing Sugar and Alcohol: If you want a healthy uterus, you must cut down on processed sugar and alcohol. Reducing your intake of these substances is crucial for supporting hormonal balance and uterine health. Drinks like soda, which are high in processed sugar, can lead to insulin resistance and inflammation. These disruptions in your system can worsen conditions such as fibroids and endometriosis (Aune et al., 2012).

Alcohol also impacts hormone levels by slowing liver function, which interferes with your body's ability to process hormones effectively. This imbalance can potentially lead to an excess of estrogen and contribute to hormone-sensitive conditions (Gavaler, 1993).

I'll admit, cutting out sugar was a real challenge for me. I loved milk chocolate and sweet milk tea, and at first, letting them go felt almost impossible. But once I committed, I felt so much lighter—both physically and energetically. My bloating reduced significantly, and I had more stable energy throughout the day. The benefits have been incredible.

Cutting Back on Red Meat: Having learned the effects of red meat on uterine health through several videos on TikTok and YouTube, I made the decision to cut back. Lamb was the hardest to let go of, but now I enjoy it only occasionally and much less frequently than before. Over time, my cravings for red meat have faded, and I've naturally started reaching for fruits and vegetables instead.

Joining a fasting support group on Discord has been a great motivator. In this group, we occasionally fast by eating only fruits and vegetables, which has kept me inspired and supported in maintaining these dietary changes. Reducing red meat intake is known to lower inflammation, benefiting reproductive health and potentially reducing the risk of fibroid growth (Peisch et al., 2017).

Personalized Nutrition: It's important to note that everyone's body is unique. What worked for me may not be the right fit for you. Before making significant changes to your diet—especially if it involves cutting out certain foods—consult with your doctor or a qualified nutritionist to ensure your choices align with your individual health needs. But one this is for certain. In all things, remain hydrated.

Hormone-Balancing Smoothie

Inspired by the hormone-balancing principles from Alisa Vitti's (Vitti, 2013):

Ingredients

1 cup organic spinach or kale

1/2 cup frozen organic berries (for antioxidants and fiber)

1 tablespoon ground organic flaxseeds (for omega-3s and hormone balance)

1/2 organic avocado (for healthy fats)

1 cup unsweetened almond milk or coconut water

Optional: 1/2 teaspoon maca powder (for added hormonal support). Blend all ingredients until smooth and joy!

CHAPTER 4

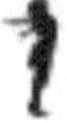

THE IMPORTANCE OF VITAMIN D

Vitamin D, often called the "sunshine vitamin," plays a crucial role in overall health. Acting as a prohormone, vitamin D supports the production of key hormones that regulate energy, mood, and general well-being (Chowdhury et al., 2017). It is especially important for balancing hormones like estrogen, which, when unbalanced, can contribute to conditions such as uterine fibroids (Paffoni et al., 2013; Baird et al., 2013).

Why Vitamin D Is Important

Hormonal Balance: Vitamin D helps balance hormones like estrogen and progesterone, which are essential for reproductive health. A deficiency can lead to hormonal imbalances, causing mood swings, fatigue, and conditions like fibroids (Baird et al., 2013).

Immune Support: Vitamin D strengthens the immune system by enhancing the pathogen-fighting effects of immune cells and reducing inflammation. A stronger immune system helps reduce fatigue and supports overall vitality (Aranow, 2011).

Cellular Energy Production: By regulating mitochondria, the energy powerhouses of cells, vitamin D ensures nutrients are efficiently converted into energy, supporting muscle function, mental clarity, and vitality (Chowdhury et al., 2017).

Reduction of Inflammation; Chronic inflammation can lead to fatigue and other low-energy symptoms. Vitamin D's anti-inflammatory properties help reduce overall inflammation (Aranow, 2011).

Mood and Mental Health: Vitamin D plays a role in producing serotonin, the "feel-good" neurotransmitter. Adequate levels can stabilize mood and may help prevent conditions like seasonal affective disorder (SAD) (Penckofer et al., 2010).

Vitamin D: A Key Player in Uterine Health

Vitamin D has been studied extensively for its role in reducing the risk and progression of uterine fibroids. Women with lower vitamin D levels are more likely to develop fibroids—non-cancerous growths in the uterus that can cause heavy bleeding, pelvic pain, and fertility challenges (Baird et al., 2013; Paffoni et al., 2013).

Research suggests that vitamin D helps prevent fibroid growth by balancing hormone levels, especially estrogen, which is closely linked to fibroid development. It also inhibits fibroid cell growth by reducing the activity of genes involved in cell proliferation. Women with sufficient vitamin D levels have been found to have up to a 32% lower risk of developing fibroids compared to those who are deficient (Baird et al., 2013).

Sunlight and Vitamin D

The most natural way to obtain vitamin D is through sunlight. When UVB rays contact the skin, they trigger vitamin D production (Holick, 2007). However, factors like skin type, geographic location, and season can affect how much sunlight is needed. For those in northern climates or with darker skin, it can be difficult to produce enough vitamin D from sunlight alone, as melanin reduces the skin's ability to synthesize vitamin D (Holick, 2004). In such cases, dietary sources or supplements are essential. Consult a healthcare provider to find the best supplement option for you.

Outdoor Tips for Boosting Your Vitamin D

Morning or Late Afternoon Sun: Aim for 15–30 minutes of sun exposure during the early morning or late afternoon to avoid harsh UV rays. People with darker skin may need more time outdoors, as melanin can reduce vitamin D synthesis (Lips, 2006; Holick, 2004).

Walks or Yoga in the Park: Combine your vitamin D boost with activities like walking, yoga, or stretching in a park or backyard. This not only supports vitamin D production but also enhances body and mental wellness.

Gardening or Outdoor Chores: Do you own a garden? Use this opportunity to tend to it with the intention of soaking up some sunshine vitamin. Gardening not only connects you to nature but also provides a wonderful way to boost your vitamin D levels while nurturing your plants and yourself.

Outdoor Workouts: Take your exercise routine outdoors. Running, bodyweight exercises, or stretching in nature can add variety to your routine while supporting vitamin D absorption. Make sure you're well-protected and choose times when the sun isn't too harsh. If possible, work out in the shade to stay cool and avoid overexposure.

Weekend Hikes or Picnics: Plan hikes or picnics to reconnect with nature and absorb vitamin D. A few hours outdoors can have lasting benefits for your body and mind.

Wear Sleeveless or Light Clothing: Opt for clothing that exposes more skin, like sleeveless tops or light dresses, to maximize sunlight absorption.

Limit Sunscreen for Short Periods: While sunscreen is essential for skin protection, it can block vitamin D production. For short periods (15–20 minutes), delay applying sunscreen to allow your skin to absorb some sun. Always avoid prolonged exposure to prevent UV damage.

If you have skin concerns, consult your doctor before limiting sunscreen use (Holick, 2007).

Vitamin D is a vital element of overall health, particularly for balancing hormones and supporting uterine well-being. By embracing sunlight and incorporating vitamin D-rich habits into your daily routine, you can take a powerful step toward achieving uterine balance, sustained energy, and overall wellness.

CHAPTER 5

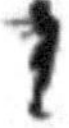

STRESS AND FIBROIDS

Did you know that it's possible for stress to affect your body in ways similar to toxins? While we often think of toxins as chemicals, pollutants, or unhealthy foods, stress can be just as harmful to your health. Left unmanaged, stress disrupts your body and causes damage that mirrors the effects of toxins.

Studies show that chronic stress triggers the release of hormones like cortisol, which can lead to inflammation, hormone imbalances, and a weakened immune system—much like toxins do. These conditions create an environment that encourages fibroid growth, something I experienced firsthand during one of my most stressful periods (Sapolsky, 2004).

Before my myomectomy, running my small business felt overwhelming. Constant worries about finances and daily tasks left me stressed, and during this time, my periods became much heavier. I didn't make the connection then, but looking back, I now realize that chronic stress was likely contributing to the growth of my fibroids and the heavy bleeding. Interestingly, many doctors don't discuss how stress affects uterine health or contributes to fibroid growth unless you ask. I stumbled upon the connection through a YouTube video and realized how much stress was influencing my body. Armed with this knowledge, I decided to flow with life and make intentional changes to reduce my stress triggers for better overall health.

Had I understood this connection earlier, I would have prioritized reducing stress and taken better care of myself to protect my uterine health. But What's done is done, and we can only look ahead. My hope is that you, the reader, will take this to heart and prioritize reducing stress in your life if it's present. Taking better care of yourself now could make all the difference.

How Stress Mirrors the Effect of Toxins on Your Body

Inflammation: Stress increases inflammation, disrupting balance in the uterus and creating conditions favorable to fibroid growth, much like external toxins disrupt other systems (Miller, Chen, & Cole, 2007).

Hormonal Imbalances: Chronic stress elevates cortisol levels, which can disrupt reproductive hormones like estrogen and progesterone. Elevated estrogen, in particular, fuels fibroid growth (Khan et al., 2014).

Immune System Suppression: Stress weakens the immune system, making it harder for the body to combat abnormal cell growth that may contribute to fibroids (Chrousos, 2009).

Oxidative Stress and Cell Damage: Stress causes oxidative stress, leading to cell damage similar to the effects of free radicals. This has been linked to fibroid progression, emphasizing the importance of stress management (Choi et al., 2010).

The Role of Cortisol and Hormonal Disruption

When the body experiences chronic stress, cortisol and adrenaline levels rise, impacting the hypothalamic-pituitary-adrenal (HPA) axis, which helps regulate hormone balance. Prolonged activation of the HPA axis can increase estrogen production, fueling fibroid growth (Matsuda et al., 2016).

Cortisol also interferes with the liver's ability to detoxify excess estrogen, further disrupting hormonal balance. This buildup of estrogen can increase the size of fibroids and worsen symptoms (Cohen & Williamson, 1991).

Stress Management as a Tool for Fibroid Relief

Given the strong connection between stress and fibroids, stress management can play a crucial role in prevention and symptom relief. Practices like mindfulness, yoga, meditation, and deep breathing help reduce cortisol levels, restore hormonal balance, and may even slow fibroid growth (Bower et al., 2015). Lowering stress also reduces inflammation, strengthening the body's resilience and improving its ability to manage fibroids.

Incorporating relaxation techniques into your daily routine can enhance well-being and minimize fibroid symptoms. Research suggests that effective stress management may lead to fewer symptoms, less pain, and slower fibroid progression (Wise et al., 2004).

Tips for a Stress-Free Day
First Hour

Meditation (10-15 minutes): Start your day with meditation or deep breathing. Focus on your breath and release any tension, especially around your lower abdomen. This activates the parasympathetic nervous system, reducing stress hormones and promoting balance.

Warm Lemon Water: Hydrate with warm lemon water to support digestion and detoxification, helping to clear out toxins that exacerbate inflammation and hormonal imbalances.

Yoga or Stretching (15-20 minutes) Incorporate movements like hip circles or child's pose to increase blood flow to the pelvic area and relieve tension.

Midday and Afternoon

Lunch: Eat a meal rich in anti-inflammatory foods, such as leafy greens, avocado, nuts, and berries. Eat mindfully to nurture your body.

Herbal Tea: Organic herbal teas like red raspberry leaf, nettle, or chamomile can calm the nervous system and support uterine health.

Nature Walk: Spend time outdoors, walking mindfully and breathing deeply. A short walk can reset your nervous system, lower cortisol levels, and leave you feeling refreshed (Park et al., 2010; Hansen et al., 2017; Bratman et al., 2012).

Journaling: Write down your thoughts and feelings to release pent-up emotions that may contribute to stress and tension.

Evening

Do Nothing. Give yourself permission to rest and recharge. Use this time to reflect, relax, or simply enjoy the moment without distractions. Reducing stress creates a healthier environment for your body.

CHAPTER 6

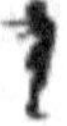

PHYSICAL MOVEMENT & WOMB HEALTH

Physical movement plays a transformative role in overall health, and its impact on womb health is especially significant. For women managing fibroids or other reproductive health concerns, incorporating movement into daily life can provide essential support for both body and mind (Baird & Dunson, 2003).

Benefits Of Physical Movement for Womb Health

Improved circulation: Physical movement boosts blood flow throughout the body, including the pelvic region where the uterus resides. Proper circulation delivers oxygen and nutrients to uterine tissue, reducing stagnation, which is often linked to fibroid growth and other reproductive issues (Wise et al., 2006).

Hormonal Balance: Exercise helps regulate hormones, particularly estrogen and progesterone, which are critical for reproductive health. Regular physical activity can reduce excess estrogen levels, aiding in the management of fibroids, endometriosis, and other uterine conditions.

Regular physical activity can lower excess estrogen levels, which is beneficial for managing fibroids, endometriosis, and other uterine conditions.

Studies suggest that women who engage in moderate to vigorous exercise have a reduced risk of developing fibroids compared to those with sedentary lifestyles (Marshall et al., 1998). Additionally, physical activity helps regulate insulin and other metabolic hormones, lowering the risk of insulin resistance—a condition linked to PCOS and fibroid growth (Velez Edwards et al., 2013).

Reduced Inflammation: Chronic inflammation is linked to many reproductive health issues, including fibroids. Activities such as aerobic exercise and yoga can lower inflammation markers in the body, easing uterine inflammation and promoting overall reproductive wellness (Calle & Thun, 2004).

Emotional Well-Being: Exercise stimulates the release of endorphins, natural mood boosters that reduce stress hormone levels (Segerstrom & Miller, 2004). Since chronic stress can exacerbate hormonal imbalances and reproductive health challenges, incorporating physical activity into your routine can provide critical emotional and physical support for your womb.

Weight Management: Maintaining a healthy weight through regular movement is vital for reproductive health. Excess weight can disrupt hormonal balance, leading to increased estrogen production, which may fuel fibroid growth. Research has shown that women with higher BMI are at greater risk of developing fibroids, making exercise a key component of womb health (Wise et al., 2005).

Exercise Ideas for Womb Health

Walking: Walking is a simple, low-impact activity that improves circulation, reduces stress, and supports over-all well-being. It also benefits kidney health by enhancing blood flow, which helps the kidneys filter waste more efficiently.

Yoga: Hip-opening poses enhance blood flow to the pelvic area, relieve tension, and promote relaxation. Fertility or womb yoga practices are especially beneficial for reproductive health.

Dancing: A fun and energizing way to get your blood flowing, relieve stress, and boost your mood.

Strength Training: Exercises like squats and lunges engage the core and pelvic floor muscles, improve metabolic health, and support hormonal balance.

Swimming: A low-impact workout that enhances cardiovascular health, builds muscle, and improves circulation to reproductive organs while promoting hormonal balance.

CHAPTER 7

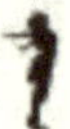

REST AND RECOVERY FOR WOMB HEALTH

Rest and recovery are vital for supporting womb health, yet in today's productivity-focused world, we have forgotten just how restorative rest can be. Giving yourself permission to slow down creates the space your body needs to reset, recharge, and truly thrive. Dedicating a day to rest isn't indulgent—it's an act of love and an investment in your well-being (Anderson et al., 2019).

Why Rest Matters for a Woman's Well-being

Hormonal Balance: Rest plays a key role in keeping hormones like estrogen and progesterone balanced, especially during menstruation when hormone levels fluctuate and energy naturally dips. Taking time to rest during your cycle can ease symptoms such as cramps and fatigue. Chronic stress and lack of sleep elevate cortisol levels, disrupting hormonal balance and potentially worsening conditions like fibroids (Matsuda et al., 2016).

Stress Reduction: Rest helps the body shift from "fight or flight" mode to "rest and digest" mode, which reduces cortisol levels. Lower cortisol supports hormonal balance and overall well-being (Segerstrom & Miller, 2004).

Reducing Inflammation: Adequate rest allows the body to release anti-inflammatory chemicals that support healing. Conversely, lack of sleep and chronic stress can increase inflammation, which negatively affects reproductive health (Irwin, Olmstead, & Carroll, 2016).

Emotional Healing: The womb is not only a physical space but also an energetic center that holds tension, emotions, and creative potential. When the body and mind are well-rested, the womb benefits deeply, nurturing emotional balance and unlocking its innate power to manifest your dreams and intentions through the practices introduced in Chapter 1. Rest creates the space needed for emotional healing and alignment, allowing you to reconnect with your inner self.

Creating A Day of Rest

Every woman deserves to dedicate at least one day a month to herself—a day to recharge, reset, and feel completely refreshed. Imagine setting aside this time to focus entirely on your well-being. Here's a simple rest routine to help your body and mind enjoy a well-deserved break:

Take an intentional Day Off for Rest- Rise naturally, without an alarm if possible. Start the day with deep breaths and stretches to set a calm and mindful tone for the day

2. ***Breakfast:*** Break your fast with a glass of pure water and a squeeze of lemon for liver health and to kick-start your metabolism.

3. ***Home Spa Day-*** Create a relaxing atmosphere with a candle or your favorite essential oils. Play soothing music, put on a face mask, and enjoy a warm bath to calm both your body and mind.

4. ***Detach from Energy Drainers-*** Avoid anything that might drain your energy. Turn off your phone, skip social media, and steer clear of stressful activities like impulse spending or watching the news. Focus on being fully present in the moment.

5. ***Eat Well-*** Prepare something wholesome and nourishing, like a sandwich with leafy greens, avocado, and quality protein, or a bowl of fresh fruits and vegetables. Eat slowly, savoring each bite as a grounding act of self-care.

6 ***Light Exercises*** While rest is the goal, gentle exercises can be beneficial. Try stretching, yoga, or a short, relaxing walk to keep your body feeling balanced and refreshed.

7. ***Get Outside for a Bit:*** Step outside to soak in fresh air and sunlight. Find a quiet spot under a tree, enjoy a few moments in the sun, or take a short, mindful walk in nature. Time spent outdoors can work wonders for your mood and energy, offering a peaceful retreat from daily

stress. Forests are for rest—let their calming energy envelop you. Bring along a good book or your favorite herbal tea to make the experience even more enjoyable and fulfilling.

8. ***Reflect and Journal*** - Take a few minutes to write down any thoughts or feelings from the day.

CHAPTER 8

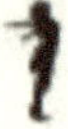

BENEFITS OF HERBAL TEAS

Herbal teas have been used for centuries to naturally support womb health and promote balance within the reproductive system. Certain herbs, when brewed into teas, offer soothing, nourishing, and healing benefits that may help manage common reproductive health concerns like fibroids, PMS, menstrual cramps, and hormonal imbalances (Clare et al., 2009; Lutgen, 2019). Let us explore a few herbal teas that can be especially beneficial for womb health.

1. Red Raspberry Leaf Tea

Organic Red raspberry leaf is one of the most well-known herbs for supporting uterine health. It's rich in vitamins and minerals like magnesium, potassium, iron, and B vitamins, all of which help strengthen the uterine muscles. This makes it particularly beneficial for women dealing with menstrual cramps or fibroids.

Benefits: Red raspberry leaf tones the uterus, alleviates heavy menstrual bleeding, and reduces menstrual cramps (McFarlin et al., 1999).

How to use*:* Drink red raspberry leaf tea daily, particularly in the second half of your menstrual cycle, to tone and support the uterus.

2. Ginger Tea

Organic Ginger is a powerful anti-inflammatory herb that can reduce pain and discomfort associated with menstrual cramps and fibroids. It also supports digestion and enhances circulation, which helps in reducing inflammation in the body.

Benefits: Ginger tea helps relieve cramps and reduces inflammation in the uterus (Omidvar & Begum, 2014).

How to use: Steep fresh ginger root in hot water for 10-15 minutes and drink it warm to ease discomfort.

3. Chamomile Tea

Organic Chamomile is well-known for its calming properties, but it also acts as an anti-inflammatory agent. Chamomile tea can help reduce stress, which is crucial because stress hormones can exacerbate hormonal imbalances, and it also helps with menstrual cramps by relaxing the muscles of the uterus.

Benefits: Chamomile relaxes the uterus, reduces stress, and promotes overall hormonal balance (Sharafzadeh et al., 2011).

How to use: Drink chamomile tea before bed to help relax and soothe the body.

4. Dandelion Root Tea

Organic Dandelion root is a wonderful herb for detoxification which helps eliminate excess estrogen from the body.

Estrogen dominance is often a factor in the development of fibroids, and dandelion root tea supports liver function, which is responsible for processing and clearing hormones from the body.

Benefits: Dandelion tea promotes liver detoxification, helps reduce estrogen dominance, and supports womb health (Clare et al., 2009).

How to use: Drink dandelion root tea in the morning to kickstart your detoxification process.

5. Nettle Tea

Organic Nettle tea is rich in nutrients that support womb health and overall wellness. Packed with iron, calcium, and magnesium, it replenishes essential nutrients, which can be especially helpful for women with heavy periods due to fibroids or other conditions. Nettle also aids in detoxification, helping to flush out toxins and promote healthy blood flow. However, if you have a thyroid condition, it's best to consult your healthcare provider before using nettle tea (Lutgen, 2019).

Benefits: Nettle tea helps with blood detoxification, boosts iron levels, and supports overall reproductive health (Lutgen, 2019). If you have underlying health conditions or thyroid issues, consult your doctor before use.

How to use: Drink nettle tea daily to nourish blood health and support the womb, especially during or after heavy periods. Always consult your doctor if you have any underlying health conditions.

6. Motherwort Tea

Organic Motherwort is a traditional herb used to support women's reproductive health. Known for its calming effect on the nervous system, it can help reduce menstrual cramps and support a balanced menstrual cycle. It's also believed to assist the uterus in returning to its normal size after pregnancy.

Benefits: Motherwort tones the uterus, regulates menstruation, and relieves menstrual cramps (Hoffmann, 2003).

How to use: Use motherwort tea during your menstrual cycle or whenever you're experiencing cramps or irregular cycles. Be sure to consult with your physician before use.

7. Hibiscus Tea

Organic Hibiscus tea is filled with antioxidants and vitamin C, supporting immune health and helping to maintain hormonal balance. It's also known for helping to regulate blood pressure, which is great for overall wellness (McKay et al., 2010). Always consult with your healthcare provider before adding it to your routine.

Benefits: Hibiscus tea promotes hormonal balance and supports liver detoxification, which can help regulate estrogen levels (Gurrola-Díaz et al., 2010).

How to use: Drink hibiscus tea regularly to maintain healthy hormone levels and support the detoxification of excess estrogen.

8. Green Tea

Organic Green tea has antioxidants that reduce inflammation and support healthy cell function. Research suggests that its anti-inflammatory and anti-proliferative properties may help shrink fibroids and inhibit their growth (Roshdy et al., 2013). Please, consult with your physician.

Benefits: Green tea may help reduce fibroid size and lower inflammation in the body (Roshdy et al., 2013).

How to use: Drink 1-2 cups of green tea daily to help reduce fibroid size and inflammation in the womb.

9. Peppermint Tea

Peppermint tea is soothing for digestive health and supports the relaxation of uterine muscles. It can alleviate cramps, bloating, and stress, which can all contribute to menstrual discomfort.

Benefits: Peppermint tea relaxes the uterus and reduces menstrual cramps (Modares et al., 2012).

How to use: Drink peppermint tea throughout your menstrual cycle to relieve cramps and to soothe the digestive system.

Tea Disclaimer

The information about these herbal teas is publicly available and shared here to support womb health. However, these teas are not a substitute for professional medical advice. Always consult with a healthcare provider for personalized guidance.

Getting the Most Herbal Teas Out of Your Teas!

Be consistent: Herbal teas work best with regular use. Try drinking one or two cups daily, depending on the herb, and observe how your body responds over time.

Rotate your herbs: Each herb offers unique benefits, so consider rotating them based on your needs in different phases of your cycle.

Consult a professional: If you have any underlying health conditions, check with a healthcare provider before adding new herbs to your routine.

CHAPTER 9

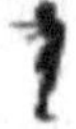

CLEAN LIVING

Cleanliness is godliness. It embodies the energy of the divine and reflects our physical, mental, and energetic states. Clean living goes beyond healthy eating or tidying up—it's about creating a lifestyle that nurtures both physical and energetic balance. When we live clean in body and spirit, we become less affected by environmental stressors. This higher frequency allows us to live peacefully and in harmony. A clean and balanced state not only supports overall well-being but also helps reduce the risk of reproductive issues like fibroids.

Physical cleanliness

Physical cleanliness is essential for helping your body thrive. By reducing exposure to toxins, maintaining proper hygiene, eating nourishing foods, and supporting natural detoxification, you create a clean, supportive environment that promotes balance and resilience especially for womb health. Here are some simple ways to incorporate physical clean living into your daily routine:

1.*Avoiding Harmful Chemicals*- Many household items, like cleaners and cosmetics, often contain chemicals that can disrupt your hormones—something essential for womb health. Ingredients like phthalates, BPA, and parabens have been linked to hormonal imbalances and reproductive concerns, including fibroid growth (Diamanti-Kandarakis et al., 2009).

Switch to natural cleaning products: Opt for organic, chemical-free alternatives in your personal care and household cleaning whenever possible. Small, simple swaps—like using baking soda and vinegar for cleaning or coconut oil as a moisturizer—can significantly reduce toxin exposure. The best part? These changes are budget-friendly and easy to incorporate into your daily routine.

2. Detoxifying Your Body*:* Caring for your body is not just about avoiding harmful substances—it's also about providing it with the right tools to cleanse and restore itself. Your diet plays a major role in this process. What you choose to eat can either nourish your body or burden it with toxins. Let's explore how to detoxify through mindful eating and hydration.

Increase fiber intake: Women should increase their intake of high-fiber foods, such as leafy greens, whole grains, and berries. These nutrient-rich options are excellent for helping the body eliminate excess estrogen, a hormone often linked to fibroid growth (Sitruk-Ware, 2006).

Stay Hydrated: Drinking enough water is essential for flushing out toxins and supporting overall health. Aim for at least 8 cups a day and try adding a squeeze of lemon to boost liver function. Hydrating fruits like watermelon, cucumbers, and oranges are also great options to keep your body balanced, refreshed, and nourished.

3.Minimize Environmental Toxins: Your environment plays a significant role in shaping your life and manifestations. Don't manifest fibroids by remaining in the wrong environment. Be mindful of your exposure to common toxins like pesticides, heavy metals, and plastics. These environmental pollutants can disrupt hormone regulation and accumulate in the body over time, potentially contributing to reproductive issues, including fibroids (Diamanti-Kandarakis et al., 2009).

Energetic Cleanliness

Maintaining an energetically balanced space is just as important as physical cleanliness. Unresolved emotions, negative influences, and clutter in your surroundings are energetic manifestations that cause imbalances, drain your mood, deplete your energy, and disrupt your sense of harmony. Caring for your energy helps create a light, positive, and peaceful environment that protects both your inner and outer balance. Here are a few simple ways to maintain energetic cleanliness and create a balanced, uplifting space.

Clearing Emotional and Energetic Blockages: Our bodies and minds often hold onto emotions, trauma, and stress, which can ultimately create energetic blockages that disrupt balance and harmony. By incorporating ancient practices like grounding, energy healing, dance, and affirmations, you can release these blockages, restore the natural flow of energy, and enhance your overall well-being.

Meditations and Visualizations: During meditation, take a deep breath and envision a warm, golden light entering your body. Feel this light flowing gently through every part of you, melting away tension, dissolving stored emotions, and clearing energetic blockages. Remember, imagination is the gateway to reality—use it to draw healing and balance into your life.

Grounding Practices for Inflammation Relief: Grounding, also known as "earthing," involves direct contact with the Earth, such as walking barefoot on grass, soil, or sand. This simple yet powerful practice helps neutralize the effects of daily exposure to electronics, which generate an excess of positive ions. Africans have understood the power of earthing for generations. Walking barefoot isn't always a sign of poverty; often, it's an instinctive connection to the Earth's healing energy. This ancestral wisdom reminds us of the restorative power of being grounded in nature.

On some occasions, you may even see an African carrying their shoes while walking barefoot. I know this because I used to do it myself without thinking much of it, but it always left me feeling amazing. Grounding restores balance by reducing inflammation, easing stress, and promoting both physical and emotional harmony (*Chevalier et al., 2015*).

Maintain an Energetically Clean Home

The energy of your home can either uplift you or weigh you down. A clean, clutter-free living space invites positive energy while nurturing your emotional and spiritual well-being. Think of cleaning as an act of self-love and energetic care, a way to honor yourself and the space you occupy.

Declutter Regularly: Cleaning allows your home to take care of you. As you clean, speak to your home with gratitude. Thank it for sheltering you, supporting your health, and creating a space of comfort and love. Say, "Thank you, my home, for being self-sustaining and for providing the maintenance and finances that take care of you and allow me to live here." This simple act of appreciation transforms cleaning into a meaningful ritual of connection, gratitude, and care.

Maintain A Positive Mind: You have the power to shape the energy that resides in your space. It starts with your mindset: **Positive mind → Positive thoughts → Positive emotions → High vibration → Positive frequency → Positive experiences.** This simple equation reflects how maintaining a positive mindset creates a feedback loop that aligns you with the outcomes you desire.

Set Healthy Boundaries: Boundaries with people, spaces, and things that drain your energy are essential to living energetically clean. Be mindful of the media you consume, as much of today's content thrives on and creates negative energy. Protect your peace by limiting time on social media and avoiding content that leaves you feeling stressed or lacking. Distance yourself from people, places, or situations that don't align with your well-being.

Love is your majority, not the exception—you are always in love. If you find yourself worrying about being harmed, it may be because you're in the frequency of unsafety. Use your emotions and intuition to guide you in choosing where and with whom to invest your energy. Surround yourself with people who already see and support your value, not those who use your energy to build their own value. Your energy and attention are sacred—invest them in what truly brings you joy.

Meditations for an Energetically Clean Field

Living with clean energy is about cultivating harmony, balance, and order in your life. A key part of this is maintaining a clear energy field. When your energy field is clean, it enhances your well-being by clearing away negativity and making you magnetic to positive experiences. It allows you to feel emotionally balanced, mentally focused, and brimming with vitality. A clean energy field is also a protective shield that keeps you grounded and centered even in the face of external stress.

It is essential to listen to your intuition when creating and maintaining a positive energy field. Your inner voice will guide you toward practices, spaces, and people that support and uplift your energy. It will also steer you away from anything that might diminish it. Trust yourself. Trust what feels right. Let your intuition lead you toward the harmony and balance you deserve.

The source of all things is like an ocean that flows through many faucets, revealing itself in countless forms. You are not limited to what you know; you are connected to an infinite well of wisdom and possibilities. Trust in this abundance as you navigate your journey.

Meditation: Dissolving Untruths

Take a deep breath in, and as you exhale, let go of any tension or resistance. Close your eyes, center yourself, and repeat the following:

Everything I believe about myself that is untrue is now dissolved.

Everything I believe about my mother, father, or family that is untrue is now dissolved.

Everything I believe about my health that is untrue is now dissolved.

Everything I believe about my home that is untrue is now dissolved.

Everything I believe about my money, opportunities, business, or job that is untrue is now dissolved.

Everything I believe about the government that is untrue is now dissolved.

Everything I believe about my life experiences that is untrue is now dissolved.

Feel the weight of these untruths dissolving like mist in the morning sun, leaving behind clarity, peace, and truth.

Traveling on a Heavy Period

Traveling during a heavy period can feel overwhelming, but with the right preparation, it can be stress-free. While it's ideal to plan trips around your cycle, unavoidable travel doesn't have to be difficult. Here's how to prepare:

Before Your Trip

Consult Your Doctor: If heavy periods are a concern, consult your doctor. They may suggest medications like tranexamic acid to manage blood flow or other tailored treatments.

Start Drinking Nettle Tea (If Approved by Your Doctor): A few days before traveling, drink nettle tea or other feminine supportive teas to replenish iron, support hormones, reduce period and reduce fatigue. Check with your doctor first to ensure it's safe alongside any medications.

Know Your Options: Research nearby hospitals or urgent care centers along your route. Save their contact information for quick access. If flying, inform the flight crew for extra assistance if needed. They can help if needed and ensure you have easy access to the restroom.

How to Pack:

High-Absorbency Menstrual Products-Pack super-absorbent products, overnight pads, menstrual cups, or discs designed for heavy flow.

Leak-Proof Liners or Period Underwear- Add liners or wear period underwear for extra protection. Disposable seat liners or blankets can offer discreet backup. Some travel-friendly period blankets are designed with waterproof backing to protect seating surfaces discreetly.

Compression Socks- Use these to improve leg circulation and reduce swelling during long trips.

Cramp management - Pack nettle, chamomile, or ginger tea bags and doctor-approved pain relievers.

Hygiene Supplies- Include unscented wipes, a towel, spare underwear, and sealable bags for used items. Wear dark, loose-fitting clothes for comfort and confidence.

Plan Rest Stops*:* Take regular breaks to stretch your legs and use the restroom.

Stay Hydrated Hydration is essential for overall health, especially during your period. Staying hydrated helps flush toxins, maintain energy levels, and reduce bloating. For an added boost, consider iron-infused water to replenish iron lost during heavy bleeding. Consult your doctor about iron supplements such as Tot'Hema or other options they may support your needs.

CHAPTER 10

EMOTIONAL HEALING

Emotional healing is a cornerstone of womb health. As we've explored in earlier chapters, the womb is not just a physical organ but an energetic center that can hold onto unprocessed emotions, traumas, and experiences. Emotions, being a form of energy, can become "stuck" in the body when they are left unprocessed, creating blockages that may impact our well-being.

During my journey with fibroids, I began to sense a deep connection between unprocessed emotions and the progression of my condition. There was a time when I felt completely overwhelmed—by stress from relationships, the demands of work, and unresolved emotional wounds from the past. It was as though these emotions were quietly taking a toll on my body.

When I finally started to acknowledge and release these emotional burdens, everything began to shift. I noticed profound improvements in both my physical and mental health. My periods became more regular, and I experienced a newfound sense of emotional clarity and balance that had eluded me for years. By my emotions and the release of them, it was done unto me.

The Connection Between Emotional Blockages and Womb Health

Scientific research supports the link between chronic stress, unresolved emotional issues, and reproductive health challenges. Emotions such as anger, fear, and grief trigger stress responses in the body, causing the release of cortisol and other stress hormones. These hormones, when persistently elevated, can disrupt the balance of reproductive hormones like estrogen and progesterone (Segerstrom & Miller, 2004). Over time, this disruption can create an environment conducive to fibroid growth and other reproductive health issues (Khan et al., 2014).

The field of psychoneuroimmunology further illuminates how emotional and psychological stress can weaken immune function and increase inflammation—both factors that contribute to the development of fibroids and other uterine conditions (Irwin et al., 2016). By addressing and releasing emotional blockages, you not only clear energetic pathways in your womb but also empower your body's natural ability to heal and restore harmony.

If you find yourself feeling overwhelmed by unresolved

emotions, consider seeking support. A therapist, counselor, or holistic health practitioner can provide valuable tools and resources to help you navigate emotional and reproductive healing.

The Impact of Emotional Healing on Womb Health

When we process and release emotional blockages, we open up pathways for energy to flow freely. This liberation of energy can lead to deeper levels of physical, emotional, and spiritual healing. Holding back emotions and energies is, in a way, a form of stinginess—an act of withholding from yourself and the world. When energy is held back, it stagnates, and stagnation cannot expand. By releasing what no longer serves you, you allow your energy to circulate and create space for growth, balance, and harmony.

Studies suggest that stress-reduction techniques, such as meditation and mindfulness, can significantly improve reproductive health and alleviate symptoms of conditions like fibroids and endometriosis (Bower et al., 2015). Letting go is an act of generosity toward yourself—it allows you to invite in healing and renewal.

A Journey Worth Taking

Healing is a journey, not a destination. The beauty of life lies in the process, and it is this process that shapes the reward, ultimately manifested in the outcome.

Each step you take to acknowledge and release emotional burdens is a step closer to balance, well-being, and wholeness. Grant yourself the gift of patience, love, and care as you navigate this process of healing. By nurturing your emotional health, you're not only supporting your womb but also embracing your inner power to cultivate a life of harmony, abundance, and fulfillment.

Remember, do not create experiences you don't want to maintain. Be mindful of the emotions you hold and release, for it shapes the reality you live in.

CHAPTER 11

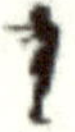

EVOCATIONS FOR HEALING AND VITALITY

We have now arrived at the part of this book where we present evocations—words of power to help you call upon healing and vitality. But what are evocations? Evocations are spoken or written invitations that summon specific energies, emotions, or intentions. They connect deeply with your spiritual and energetic essence, allowing you to manifest the energy you wish to embody.

You might be wondering, what's the difference between evocations and affirmations? While affirmations focus on reinforcing personal beliefs or mindsets, evocations go deeper. They transcend the personal and connect with the collective spiritual, emotional, and energetic realms, inviting powerful energies to align with your intentions.

In this section, the evocations are aligned with specific topics, Remember, the material realm is the final stage of creation, while the mental realm is where it all begins. In the mental space, thoughts take shape and intentions are set, laying the foundation for what manifests in the physical world. Your words hold immense power in this unseen realm of creation. Who are you in consciousness?

We have no beginning, and we have no end. We, as creation, come into being wherever consciousness permits. We awaken when consciousness deems us ready. Speaking evocations builds the energy needed to move toward an awakened state of your desired reality. Use these evocations as tools to align with higher consciousness and unlock your infinite potential. So, let's begin.

Evocation For Love and Healing

I am presently aware of the infinite love and healing energy that surrounds me. I am in a world that loves and heals me, and I open my heart to receive its blessings. I am held in love, nourished by healing, and uplifted by the divine energy that flows through all things. Love and healing are my constant companions, and I embrace them fully in every moment.

Evocation For Understanding My Body

I call upon the divine wisdom within to deepen my understanding of my body. I honor my body's sacred messages and trust the truths it reveals to me. I trust my body's intelligence and its infinite power to heal. With gratitude, I receive the guidance my body so lovingly provides.

Evocation For the Energy of Vitamin D

I call upon the sunshine vitamin within me. I am deeply connected to the healing power of the sun and all of nature, for I know we come from one source. As I spend time in the sun, my body absorbs its radiant energy, renewing my strength and vitality. I am grateful for the sunlight that helps generate the healthy foods I eat. My cells are vibrant, healthy, and brimming with life. I am nourished, empowered, and harmonized with the vitality of the universe.

Evocation for Healthy Eating

I call upon my body's wisdom to guide me toward foods that nourish and heal. I am in tune with my body's needs, and today, I choose what truly enriches my well-being. My eating habits honor and support the sacred connection between food and healing.

Evacuation for Herbal Teas for Womb Health

I welcome the healing energy of herbal teas. Each herb carries the Earth's healing wisdom. With every sip, my uterus is healed and supported by these natural remedies. I am filled with vibrant, balanced energy. I am grateful for the generous and loving gifts of the Earth.

Evocation For Dealing with Stress

I call upon the divine power within me to release all known and unknown burdens of stress and tension. I invite my awareness to align with the deep peace that resides within me. My mind and body are spaces of pure serenity and joy. I trust my body's natural ability to heal and guide me forward. I now move through life with ease, peace, and abundant grace.

Evocation For Physical Movement

I call forth the sacred energy that animates my being. Every movement creates energy and vibrancy within me. My life force moves freely. It brings strength, renewal, and balance to every part of my body. Exercise removes blocks and allows energy to flow effortlessly. Movement restores my entire being. I am energized. I am empowered. I am in harmony with the rhythm of life. I gladly welcome the rewards of physical movement.

Evocation for Rest and Restoration

I honor the power of rest and the renewal it brings. My body knows how to heal and restore itself in every way. With each moment of rest, I let go of tension and welcome peace. I feel refreshed, whole, and calm. Rest gives me the energy I need, and I embrace it as an act of love and care for myself.

Evocation for Physical and Energetic Cleanliness

I welcome the energy of purity into my body, mind, and spirit. My surroundings are safe, clean, and supportive. I thrive in a space filled with positive energy. As I clean my home, I release stagnant energy and invite fresh, uplifting vibrations. I let go of everything that no longer serves me. My energy field is clear, vibrant, and aligned with my highest good. From this moment, I attract only energies that uplift and empower me. I am grateful for my home. It sustains and supports my journey to health and harmony.

Evocation For the Awareness of Beauty

I see beauty in all its forms. Life has opened my eyes to the beauty of health, wellness, and abundance. I align with this beauty. I know it is already within me. I radiate beauty. I express and manifest beauty in every space and every timeline. Beauty surrounds me. Beauty flows through me effortlessly. I am beauty-full.

Evocation for Gratitude

I am eternally grateful for the complete and holistic wellness within me. My body, mind, and spirit are aligned in perfect harmony, and I honor this balance with deep gratitude. My womb is a sacred space of joy, health, and creativity, and I give thanks for its vitality. I am whole, I am healed, and I radiate the energy of life. And so, it is.

REFERENCES

Afua, Q. (2001). Sacred Woman: A Guide to Healing the Feminine Body, Mind, and Spirit. One World/Ballantine.

Kent, T. L. (2011). Wild Feminine: Finding Power, Spirit & Joy in the Female Body. Atria Books/Beyond Words.

Northrup, C. (2010). Women's Bodies, Women's Wisdom: Creating Physical and Emotional Health and Healing. Bantam

References 2

Baird, D. D., & Patisaul, H. B. (2021). Environmental endocrine disruptors and fibroid risk. Environmental Health Perspectives, 129(7), 077004.

Parker, W. H. (2007). Etiology, symptomatology, and diagnosis of uterine myomas. Fertility and Sterility, 87(4), 725-736.

Stewart, E. A. (2015). Clinical practice. Uterine fibroids. The New England Journal of Medicine, 372(17), 1646-1655.

Taylor, M., & Parrott, E. (2023). The role of MED12 gene mutations in the development of uterine fibroids. Journal of Reproductive Medicine, 68(2), 102-110.

U.S. Department of Health and Human Services. (2024). Uterine fibroids fact sheet. Office on Women's Health. Retrieved from https://www.womenshealth.gov

Vollenhoven, B. J. (1998). Introduction: The epidemiology of uterine fibroids. Baillière's Clinical Obstetrics and Gynaecology, 12(2), 169-176.

References 3

Aune, D., Chan, D. S., Vieira, A. R., Navarro Rosenblatt, D. A., Vieira, R., Greenwood, D. C., & Norat, T. (2012). Dietary sugar intake and cancer risk: Results from the EPIC cohort. Annals of

Oncology, 23(10), 2610-2618.

Breymeyer, K. L., Lampe, J. W., McGregor, B. A., & Neuhouser, M. L. (2016). Subjective improvements in mood and mental clarity after reducing dietary sugar intake. Nutritional Neuroscience, 19(10), 497-504.

David, L. A., et al. (2014). Diet rapidly and reproducibly alters the human gut microbiome. Nature, 505(7484), 559-563. This study discusses how dietary changes, including sugar intake, impact gut bacteria, digestion, and bloating.

Benton, D., & Young, H. A. (2015). Reducing sugar intake may help stabilize energy levels. Nutrients, 7(1), 529-548. This review covers the impact of sugar on blood glucose and energy levels.

Gavaler, J. S. (1993). Alcoholic beverages as a source of estrogens. Alcohol Health and Research World, 17(2), 137-143.

Missmer, S. A., Chavarro, J. E., Malspeis, S., Rich-Edwards, J. W., Willett, W. C., & Hankinson, S. E. (2004). A prospective study of dietary fat consumption and endometriosis risk. Human Reproduction, 19(8), 1778-1783.

Peisch, S. F., Van Blarigan, E. L., Chan, J. M., Stampfer, M. J., & Kenfield, S. A. (2017). Prostate cancer progression and mortality: A review of diet and lifestyle factors. World Journal of Urology, 35(6), 867-874.

Smith-Spangler, C., Brandeau, M. L., Hunter, G. E., Bavinger, J. C., Pearson, M., Eschbach, P. J., ... & Bravata, D. M. (2012). Are organic foods safer or healthier than conventional alternatives?: A systematic review. Annals of Internal Medicine, 157(5), 348-366.

U.S. Department of Agriculture. (2023). Organic Standards. USDA. Retrieved from https://www.usda.gov

Vitti, A. (2013). WomanCode: Perfect Your Cycle, Amplify Your

Fertility, Supercharge Your Sex Drive, and Become a Power Source. HarperOne.

References 4

Aranow, C. (2011). Vitamin D and the immune system. Journal of Investigative Medicine, 59(6), 881-886.

Baird, D. D., Hill, M. C., Schectman, J. M., & Hollis, B. W. (2013). Vitamin D and the risk of uterine fibroids. Epidemiology, 24(3), 447-453.

Chowdhury, R., Kunutsor, S., Vitezova, A., Oliver-Williams, C., Chowdhury, S., Kiefte-de Jong, J. C., ... & Franco, O. H. (2017). Vitamin D and risk of cause-specific death: Systematic review and meta-analysis of observational cohort and randomized intervention studies. BMJ, 348, g1903.

Holick, M. F. (2004). Vitamin D: Importance in the prevention of cancers, type 1 diabetes, heart disease, and osteoporosis. American Journal of Clinical Nutrition, 79(3), 362-371.

Holick, M. F. (2007). Vitamin D deficiency. New England Journal of Medicine, 357(3), 266-281.

Lips, P. (2006). Vitamin D physiology. Progress in Biophysics and Molecular Biology, 92(1), 4-8.

Paffoni, A., Somigliana, E., Vigano, P., Benaglia, L., Vercellini, P., & Fedele, L. (2013). Vitamin D status in women with uterine leio-myomas. Journal of Clinical Endocrinology & Metabolism, 98(8), E1374-E1378.

Penckofer, S., Kouba, J., Byrn, M., & Ferrans, C. E. (2010). Vitamin D and depression: Where is all the sunshine? Issues in Mental Health Nursing, 31(6), 385-393

References 5

Bower, J. E., Low, C. A., Moskowitz, J. T., Sepah, S., Epel, E., &

Tamagawa, R. (2015). Inflammation and its mediation by stress as a potential cause of fatigue and depressive symptoms in breast cancer patients. Psychoneuroendocrinology, 37(9), 1249-1257.

Bratman, G. N., Hamilton, J. P., Hahn, K. S., Daily, G. C., & Gross, J. J. (2012). Nature experience reduces rumination and subgenual prefrontal cortex activation. Proceedings of the National Academy of Sciences, 112(28), 8567-8572.

Choi, K. H., Kim, S., & Han, J. (2010). Oxidative stress and antioxidant therapy in the progression of uterine fibroids. Free Radical Biology and Medicine, 49(6), 879-885.

Chrousos, G. P. (2009). Stress and disorders of the stress system. Nature Reviews Endocrinology, 5(7), 374-381.

Cohen, S., & Williamson, G. M. (1991). Stress and infectious disease in humans. Psychological Bulletin, 109(1), 5-24.

Hansen, M. M., Jones, R., & Tocchini, K. (2017). Shinrin-yoku (forest bathing) and nature therapy: A state-of-the-art review. International Journal of Environmental Research and Public Health, 14(8), 851.

Khan, A. T., Shehmar, M., & Gupta, J. K. (2014). Uterine fibroids: Current perspectives. International Journal of Women's Health, 6, 95-114.

Matsuda, M., Tsutsumi, K., Matsuda, T., & Kubo, Y. (2016). Cortisol and fibroid growth: Understanding the role of stress. Journal of Clinical Endocrinology and Metabolism, 101(7), 2552-2560.

Miller, G. E., Chen, E., & Cole, S. W. (2007). Health psychology: Developing biologically plausible models linking the social world and physical health. Annual Review of Psychology, 60, 501-524.

Park, B. J., Tsunetsugu, Y., Kasetani, T., Kagawa, T., & Miyazaki, Y. (2010). The physiological effects of Shinrin-yoku (taking in the forest atmosphere or forest bathing): Evidence from field experiments in 24 forests across Japan. Environmental Health and Preventive Medicine, 15(1), 18-26.

Sapolsky, R. M. (2004). Why Zebras Don't Get Ulcers: The Acclaimed Guide to Stress, Stress-Related Diseases, and Coping. Holt Paperbacks.

Wise, L. A., Palmer, J. R., Harlow, B. L., & Rosenberg, L. (2004). Reproductive factors, hormonal contraception, and risk of uterine leiomyomata in African-American women: A prospective study. American Journal of Epidemiology, 159(2), 113-123.

Reference 6

Baird, D. D., & Dunson, D. B. (2003). Why is parity protective for uterine fibroids? Epidemiology, 14(2), 247-250.

Calle, E. E., & Thun, M. J. (2004). Obesity and cancer. Oncogene, 23(38), 6365-6378.

Marshall, L. M., Spiegelman, D., Goldman, M. B., Manson, J. E., Colditz, G. A., Barbieri, R. L., ... & Hunter, D. J. (1998). A prospective study of reproductive factors and oral contraceptive use in relation to the risk of uterine leiomyomata. Fertility and Sterility, 70(3), 432-439.

Segerstrom, S. C., & Miller, G. E. (2004). Psychological stress and the human immune system: A meta-analytic study of 30 years of inquiry. Psychological Bulletin, 130(4), 601-630.

Velez Edwards, D. R., Baird, D. D., Hartmann, K. E., & Savitz, D. A. (2013). Racial differences in the prevalence of uterine leiomyomas and pelvic pain. American Journal of Obstetrics and Gynecology, 208(2), 136.e1-136.e10.

Wise, L. A., Palmer, J. R., Spiegelman, D., Harlow, B. L., Stewart, E. A., & Rosenberg, L. (2005). Influence of body size and body fat distribution on risk of uterine leiomyomata in US black women. Epidemiology, 16(3), 346-354.

Wise, L. A., Palmer, J. R., Rosenberg, L., & Harlow, B. L. (2006). Reproductive factors, hormonal contraception, and risk of uterine leiomyomata in African-American women: A prospective study. American Journal of Epidemiology, 159(2), 113-123.

References 7

Anderson, J. W., Liu, C., & Kryscio, R. J. (2019). Benefits of rest and relaxation for women's health. Journal of Women's Health, 28(5), 639-645.

Irwin, M. R., Olmstead, R., & Carroll, J. E. (2016). Sleep disturbance, sleep duration, and inflammation: A systematic review and meta-analysis of cohort studies and experimental sleep deprivation. Biological Psychiatry, 80(1), 40-52.

Matsuda, M., Tsutsumi, K., Matsuda, T., & Kubo, Y. (2016). Cortisol and fibroid growth: Understanding the role of stress. Journal of Clinical Endocrinology and Metabolism, 101(7), 2552-2560.

Segerstrom, S. C., & Miller, G. E. (2004). Psychological stress and the human immune system: A meta-analytic study of 30 years of inquiry. Psychological Bulletin, 130(4), 601-630.

References 8

Clare, B. A., Conroy, R. S., & Spelman, K. (2009). The diuretic effect in human subjects of an extract of Taraxacum officinale folium over a single day. Journal of Alternative and Complementary Medicine, 15(8), 929-934.

Gurrola-Díaz, C. M., García-López, P. M., Sánchez-Enríquez, S., Troyo-Sanromán, R., Andrade-González, I., & Gómez-Leyva, J. F. (2010). Effects of hibiscus sabdariffa on obesity in an animal model. Plant Foods for Human Nutrition, 65(4), 375-380.

Hoffmann, D. (2003). Medical Herbalism: The Science and Practice of Herbal Medicine. Healing Arts Press.

Lutgen, P. (2019). Nettle and the Healing Power of Plants: Natural Remedies for Women's Health. Health Education Publications.

McFarlin, B. L., Gibson, M. H., O'Rear, J., & Harman, P. (1999). A national survey of herbal preparation use by nurse-midwives for labor stimulation. Review of Obstetrics and Gynecology, 175(3 Pt 1), 811-816.

McKay, D. L., Chen, C. O., Saltzman, E., & Blumberg, J. B. (2010). Hibiscus sabdariffa L. tea (tisane) lowers blood pressure in prehypertensive and mildly hypertensive adults. Journal of Nutrition, 140(2), 298-303.

Modares, M., Rezaei, M., & Fahami, F. (2012). Comparison of the effect of peppermint and mefenamic acid on primary dysmenorrhea. Iranian Journal of Nursing and Midwifery Research, 17(Suppl1), S45-S49.

Omidvar, S., & Begum, K. (2014). Effectiveness of ginger in the management of primary dysmenorrhea: A systematic review and meta-analysis. Journal of Alternative and Complementary Medicine, 20(8), 657-664.

Roshdy, E., Rajaratnam, V., Maitra, S., Sabry, M., & Allah, A. S. (2013). Treatment of symptomatic uterine fibroids with green tea extract: A pilot randomized controlled clinical study. International Journal of Women's Health, 5, 477-486.

Sharafzadeh, S., Alizadeh, O., & Mashayekhi, K. (2011). Chamomile: Cultivation, processing, utilization and benefits. Journal of Medicinal Plants Research, 5(26), 5796-5800.

References 9

Chevalier, G., Sinatra, S. T., Oschman, J. L., & Delany, R. M.

(2015). Earthing (grounding) the human body reduces blood viscosity—a major factor in cardiovascular disease. Journal of Alternative and Complementary Medicine, 19(2), 102-110.

Diamanti-Kandarakis, E., Bourguignon, J. P., Giudice, L. C., Hauser, R., Prins, G. S., Soto, A. M., Zoeller, R. T., & Gore, A. C. (2009). Endocrine-disrupting chemicals: An Endocrine Society scientific statement. Endocrine Reviews, 30(4), 293-342.

Sitruk-Ware, R. (2006). New progestagens for contraceptive use. Human Reproduction Update, 12(2), 169-178.

References 10

Bower, J. E., Low, C. A., Moskowitz, J. T., Sepah, S., Epel, E., & Tamagawa, R. (2015). Inflammation and its mediation by stress as a potential cause of fatigue and depressive symptoms in breast cancer patients. Psychoneuroendocrinology, 37(9), 1249-1257.

ABOUT THE AUTHOR

I am driven by a love for the mysteries of the universe and the connections between body, mind, and spirit, I write to honor both the seen and unseen. My work's intention is to invite readers to explore, grow, and connect with their own divinity.

Thank you.

68

www.ingramcontent.com/pod-product-compliance
Lightning Source LLC
Chambersburg PA
CBHW031225160726

47992CB00006B/2895